The Joy of Healthy Eating

Delicious Recipes for a Nutritious Diet

Emma Lachance

Table of Contents:

Introduction

Eating a healthy diet is essential for overall health and well-being. A healthy diet can help you maintain a healthy weight, reduce your risk of chronic diseases, and improve your mood and energy levels.

However, eating healthy doesn't have to be boring or tasteless. In fact, there are many delicious and satisfying ways to eat a healthy diet.

This book is designed to help you enjoy the joy of healthy eating. It provides a comprehensive overview of healthy eating, including the importance of eating a variety of foods, the benefits of fruits, vegetables, and whole grains, and the role of healthy fats and proteins.

The book also includes a lot of delicious and nutritious recipes that will help you make healthy eating a part of your everyday life.

The Importance of Healthy Eating

A healthy diet is essential for overall health and well-being. Eating a healthy diet can help you:

- Maintain a healthy weight

- Reduce your risk of chronic diseases, such as heart disease, stroke, type 2 diabetes, and some types of cancer
- Improve your mood and energy levels
- Boost your immune system
- Improve your sleep

The Basics of Healthy Eating

A healthy diet is based on a variety of foods from all food groups. The five food groups are:

- Fruits
- Vegetables
- Whole grains
- Lean protein
- Healthy fats

Planning Healthy Meals

Planning healthy meals can help you make healthy choices and stick to your goals. Here are some tips for planning healthy meals:

- Choose a variety of foods from all food groups.
- Focus on whole, unprocessed foods.
- Limit processed foods, sugary drinks, and unhealthy fats.
- Cook at home more often.

Recipes

This book includes a lot of delicious and nutritious recipes that will help you make healthy eating a part of your everyday life. The recipes are organized by meal and include breakfast, lunch, dinner, and snacks.

The recipes are also labeled with nutritional information, so you can easily track your intake.

Conclusion

Eating a healthy diet is a lifelong commitment. But it doesn't have to be difficult or boring. With a little planning and effort, you can enjoy the joy of healthy eating.

Chapter 1: The Importance of Healthy Eating

Eating a healthy diet is essential for overall health and well-being. A healthy diet can help you maintain a healthy weight, reduce your risk of chronic diseases, and improve your mood and energy levels.

The Benefits of Eating a Healthy Diet

There are many benefits to eating a healthy diet, including:

- **Weight management:** Eating a healthy diet can help you maintain a healthy weight. This is important because being overweight or obese is a risk factor for many chronic diseases, such as heart disease, stroke, type 2 diabetes, and some types of cancer.

- **Reduced risk of chronic diseases:** Eating a healthy diet can help reduce your risk of developing chronic diseases. This is because a healthy diet provides your body with the nutrients it needs to function properly. Chronic diseases such as heart disease, stroke, type 2 diabetes, and some types of cancer are the leading causes of death worldwide. Eating a healthy diet can help reduce your risk of developing these diseases.

- **Improved mood and energy levels:** Eating a healthy diet can help improve your mood and energy levels. This is because a healthy diet provides your body with the nutrients it needs to produce neurotransmitters, which are chemicals that regulate mood and energy levels.

- **Boosted immune system:** Eating a healthy diet can help boost your immune system. This is important because a strong immune system helps your body fight off infection.

- **Improved sleep:** Eating a healthy diet can help improve your sleep. This is because a healthy diet provides your body with the nutrients it needs to produce melatonin, a hormone that helps regulate sleep.

The Basics of a Healthy Diet

A healthy diet is based on a variety of foods from all food groups. The five food groups are:

- **Fruits:** Fruits are a good source of vitamins, minerals, and fiber. They are also low in calories and fat.

- **Vegetables:** Vegetables are another good source of vitamins, minerals, and fiber. They are also low in calories and fat.

- **Whole grains:** Whole grains are a good source of fiber, vitamins, and minerals. They are also a good source of complex carbohydrates, which provide your body with sustained energy.

- **Lean protein:** Lean protein is a good source of protein, which is essential for building and repairing tissue.

- **Healthy fats:** Healthy fats are a good source of essential fatty acids, which are important for your health.

How to Eat a Healthy Diet

Here are some tips for eating a healthy diet:

- **Choose a variety of foods from all food groups.** This will help you ensure that you are getting all the nutrients you need.

- **Focus on whole, unprocessed foods.** Whole foods are more nutritious than processed foods.

- **Limit processed foods, sugary drinks, and unhealthy fats.** These foods are high in calories, unhealthy fats, and added sugars.

- **Cook at home more often.** This will help you control the ingredients in your food.

Conclusion

Eating a healthy diet is a lifelong commitment. But it doesn't have to be difficult or boring. With a little planning and effort, you can enjoy the joy of healthy eating.

Key Takeaways

- Eating a healthy diet is essential for overall health and well-being.
- A healthy diet can help you maintain a healthy weight, reduce your risk of chronic diseases, and improve your mood and energy levels.
- A healthy diet is based on a variety of foods from all food groups.
- Here are some tips for eating a healthy diet:
    - Choose a variety of foods from all food groups.
    - Focus on whole, unprocessed foods.

- Limit processed foods, sugary drinks, and unhealthy fats.
  - Cook at home more often.

Additional Information

- **The Centers for Disease Control and Prevention (CDC)** provides a wealth of information on healthy eating, including tips for making healthy choices, recipes, and resources for overcoming challenges.
- **The Academy of Nutrition and Dietetics** is a professional organization for registered dietitians and nutrition professionals. They offer a variety of resources on healthy eating, including fact sheets, articles, and recipes.
- **The World Health Organization (WHO)** has a global initiative to promote healthy eating and physical activity. They offer a variety of resources on healthy eating, including fact sheets, articles, and recipes.

I hope this chapter is informative and helpful.

Chapter 2: The Basics of Healthy Eating

A healthy diet is based on a variety of foods from all food groups. The five food groups are:

- **Fruits:** Fruits are a good source of vitamins, minerals, and fiber. They are also low in calories and fat.
- **Vegetables:** Vegetables are another good source of vitamins, minerals, and fiber. They are also low in calories and fat.
- **Whole grains:** Whole grains are a good source of fiber, vitamins, and minerals. They are also a good source of complex carbohydrates, which provide your body with sustained energy.
- **Lean protein:** Lean protein is a good source of protein, which is essential for building and repairing tissue.
- **Healthy fats:** Healthy fats are a good source of essential fatty acids, which are important for your health.

How to Eat a Healthy Diet

Here are some tips for eating a healthy diet:

- **Choose a variety of foods from all food groups.** This will help you ensure that you are getting all the nutrients you need.
- **Focus on whole, unprocessed foods.** Whole foods are more nutritious than processed foods.
- **Limit processed foods, sugary drinks, and unhealthy fats.** These foods are high in calories, unhealthy fats, and added sugars.
- **Cook at home more often.** This will help you control the ingredients in your food.

The Importance of Each Food Group

- **Fruits:** Fruits are a good source of vitamins, minerals, and fiber. They are also low in calories and fat. Fruits are a good source of antioxidants, which can help protect your cells from damage. They are also a good source of dietary fiber, which can help keep you feeling full and regular.
- **Vegetables:** Vegetables are another good source of vitamins, minerals, and fiber. They are also low in calories and fat. Vegetables are a good source of antioxidants, which can help protect your cells from damage. They are also a good source of dietary fiber, which can help keep you feeling full and regular.

- **Whole grains:** Whole grains are a good source of fiber, vitamins, and minerals. They are also a good source of complex carbohydrates, which provide your body with sustained energy. Whole grains are a good source of fiber, which can help keep you feeling full and regular. They are also a good source of B vitamins, which are important for energy metabolism.
- **Lean protein:** Lean protein is a good source of protein, which is essential for building and repairing tissue. Lean protein can come from a variety of sources, such as chicken, fish, beans, and tofu. Lean protein is a good source of protein, which is essential for building and repairing tissue. It is also a good source of iron, which is important for red blood cell production.
- **Healthy fats:** Healthy fats are a good source of essential fatty acids, which are important for your health. Healthy fats can come from a variety of sources, such as nuts, seeds, and avocados. Healthy fats are important for brain development and function, as well as for heart health.

Making Healthy Choices

When making food choices, it is important to choose foods that are high in nutrients and low in calories, unhealthy fats, and added sugars. Here are some tips for making healthy choices:

- **Choose fruits and vegetables over processed foods.** Fruits and vegetables are naturally low in calories and fat and high in nutrients.
- **Choose whole grains over refined grains.** Whole grains are a good source of fiber, vitamins, and minerals.
- **Choose lean protein over red meat.** Lean protein is a good source of protein without the unhealthy fats found in red meat.
- **Choose healthy fats over unhealthy fats.** Healthy fats are a good source of essential fatty acids, while unhealthy fats can raise your cholesterol levels.
- **Limit sugary drinks.** Sugary drinks are high in calories and added sugars, which can contribute to weight gain and other health problems.

Making Healthy Changes

Making healthy changes to your diet can be challenging, but it is important to remember that it is a journey, not a destination. Here are some tips for making healthy changes:

- **Start small.** Don't try to change too much at once. Start by making one or two small changes, such as adding a serving of fruits or vegetables to your meals or snacks.
- **Be patient.** It takes time to make lasting changes to your diet. Don't get discouraged if you slip up. Just keep trying.
- **Find support.** Having friends or family members who are also trying to make healthy changes can help you stay motivated.

Conclusion

Eating a healthy diet is important for overall health and well-being.

RECIPES

- **Fruit salad**
- **Yogurt parfait**
- **Oatmeal cookie**
- **Chocolate mousse**
- **Peanut butter and banana sandwich**

Fruit salad

This is a classic healthy dessert that is both delicious and refreshing. Simply combine your favorite fruits in a bowl and enjoy. You can add a dollop of yogurt or low-fat whipped cream for extra richness.

Ingredients:

- 1 cup (225g) mixed fruit, such as strawberries, blueberries, raspberries, and bananas
- 1/4 cup (60ml) plain yogurt
- 1/4 cup (60ml) low-fat whipped cream
- Honey or maple syrup, to taste

Instructions:

1. In a bowl, combine the fruit, yogurt, and whipped cream.
2. Drizzle with honey or maple syrup, to taste.
3. Serve immediately.

Yogurt parfait

This is a quick and easy dessert that is packed with nutrients. Simply layer your favorite yogurt, fruit, and granola in a glass or bowl. You can also add nuts or seeds for extra protein and healthy fats.

Ingredients:

- 1 cup (225g) plain yogurt
- 1/2 cup (120ml) fruit, such as strawberries, blueberries, or raspberries
- 1/4 cup (40g) granola
- Nuts or seeds, to taste

Instructions:

1. In a glass or bowl, layer the yogurt, fruit, granola, and nuts or seeds.
2. Serve immediately.

Oatmeal cookie

This cookie is made with whole-wheat oats, almond butter, and honey. It's a great way to get your daily dose of fiber and protein. You can also add chocolate chips or nuts for extra flavor.

Ingredients:

- 1 cup (125g) whole-wheat oats
- 1/2 cup (113g) almond butter
- 1/4 cup (60ml) honey
- 1 egg
- 1 teaspoon vanilla extract
- 1/2 teaspoon baking soda
- 1/4 teaspoon salt
- Chocolate chips or nuts, for topping (optional)

Instructions:

1. Preheat oven to 350 degrees F (175 degrees C).
2. In a large bowl, combine the oats, almond butter, honey, egg, and vanilla extract.
3. In a separate bowl, whisk together the baking soda and salt.
4. Add the dry ingredients to the wet ingredients and mix until just combined.
5. Stir in the chocolate chips or nuts, if using.
6. Drop by rounded tablespoons onto ungreased baking sheets.
7. Bake for 10-12 minutes, or until golden brown.
8. Let cool on baking sheets for a few minutes before transferring to a wire rack to cool completely.

Chocolate mousse

This mousse is made with avocados, cocoa powder, and maple syrup. It's a delicious and decadent treat that is also healthy. You can also add berries or whipped cream for extra sweetness.

Ingredients:

- 2 ripe avocados
- 1/4 cup (60ml) cocoa powder
- 1/4 cup (60ml) maple syrup
- 1/4 cup (60ml) milk
- Berries or whipped cream, for topping (optional)

Instructions:

1. In a blender, combine the avocados, cocoa powder, maple syrup, and milk.
2. Blend until smooth.
3. Pour into serving bowls or glasses.
4. Top with berries or whipped cream, if using.
5. Serve immediately.

Peanut butter and banana sandwich

This sandwich is a classic snack that is also a great dessert. Simply spread peanut butter on two slices of whole-wheat bread and top with a banana. You can also add honey or chocolate chips for extra sweetness.

Ingredients:

- 2 slices whole-wheat bread
- 1 tablespoon peanut butter
- 1/2 banana
- Honey or chocolate chips, for topping (optional)

Instructions:

1. Spread the peanut butter on one slice of bread.
2. Top with the banana.
3. Spread the peanut butter on the other slice of bread.
4. Cut in half and enjoy

Chapter 3: Planning Healthy Meals

Planning healthy meals can help you make healthy choices and stick to your goals. Here are some tips for planning healthy meals:

- **Choose a variety of foods from all food groups.** This will help you ensure that you are getting all the nutrients you need.
- **Focus on whole, unprocessed foods.** Whole foods are more nutritious than processed foods.
- **Limit processed foods, sugary drinks, and unhealthy fats.** These foods are high in calories, unhealthy fats, and added sugars.
- **Cook at home more often.** This will help you control the ingredients in your food.

How to Plan Healthy Meals

There are a few things to keep in mind when planning healthy meals:

- **Think about your goals.** What are you trying to achieve with your diet? Are you trying to lose weight, gain muscle, or improve your overall health?

- **Consider your lifestyle.** How much time do you have to cook? Do you have any dietary restrictions?
- **Make a list of your favorite foods.** This will help you choose foods that you enjoy and are likely to stick to.
- **Plan your meals for the week.** This will help you stay organized and make sure that you have everything you need on hand.
- **Be flexible.** Don't be afraid to change your plans if you need to.

Here are some examples of healthy meals:

- **Breakfast:** Oatmeal with fruit and nuts, yogurt with granola and berries, eggs with whole-wheat toast
- **Lunch:** Salad with grilled chicken or fish, soup and whole-wheat bread, whole-wheat wrap with vegetables and hummus
- **Dinner:** Grilled salmon with roasted vegetables, chicken stir-fry with brown rice, lentil soup
- **Snacks:** Fruits, vegetables, nuts, seeds

Tips for Making Healthy Meals More Enjoyable

Here are some tips for making healthy meals more enjoyable:

- **Get creative with your recipes.** There are many healthy recipes available online and in cookbooks. Experiment with different flavors and ingredients to find what you enjoy.
- **Make mealtime a social experience.** Eat with friends or family to make mealtime more enjoyable.
- **Don't be afraid to indulge sometimes.** It's okay to have a treat every once in a while. Just make sure to balance it out with healthy choices.

Conclusion

Planning healthy meals can be a challenge, but it is important for overall health and well-being. By following these tips, you can make it easier to plan and enjoy healthy meals.

RECIPES

- **Oatmeal**
- **Whole-wheat pancakes**
- **Whole-wheat waffles**
- **Whole-wheat muffins**
- **Whole-wheat bread pudding**

Oatmeal

This is a classic breakfast food that can also be enjoyed as a dessert. Simply cook oatmeal according to package directions and top with your favorite fruit, nuts, or seeds.

Ingredients:

- 1 cup (225g) rolled oats
- 2 cups (450ml) water or milk
- 1/2 teaspoon salt
- 1/4 cup (60ml) fruit, nuts, or seeds, for topping (optional)

Instructions:

1. In a medium saucepan, combine the oats, water or milk, and salt.

2. Bring to a boil, then reduce heat and simmer for 5-10 minutes, or until the oats are cooked through.
3. Serve immediately, topped with your favorite fruit, nuts, or seeds.

Whole-wheat pancakes

These pancakes are made with whole-wheat flour, which gives them a heartier texture and flavor. They're also lower in calories and fat than traditional pancakes.

Ingredients:

- 1 cup (125g) whole-wheat flour
- 1 teaspoon baking powder
- 1/2 teaspoon baking soda
- 1/4 teaspoon salt
- 1 egg
- 1 cup (240ml) milk
- 1 tablespoon oil

Instructions:

1. In a large bowl, whisk together the flour, baking powder, baking soda, and salt.
2. In a separate bowl, whisk together the egg, milk, and oil.

3. Add the wet ingredients to the dry ingredients and whisk until just combined.
4. Heat a large skillet or griddle over medium heat.
5. Pour 1/4 cup of batter onto the hot skillet for each pancake.
6. Cook for 2-3 minutes per side, or until golden brown.
7. Serve immediately.

Whole-wheat waffles

These waffles are made with whole-wheat flour, which gives them a heartier texture and flavor. They're also lower in calories and fat than traditional waffles.

Ingredients:

- 1 cup (125g) whole-wheat flour
- 1 teaspoon baking powder
- 1/2 teaspoon baking soda
- 1/4 teaspoon salt
- 1 egg
- 1 cup (240ml) milk
- 1 tablespoon oil

Instructions:

1. In a large bowl, whisk together the flour, baking powder, baking soda, and salt.
2. In a separate bowl, whisk together the egg, milk, and oil.
3. Add the wet ingredients to the dry ingredients and whisk until just combined.
4. Pour the batter into a preheated waffle iron and cook according to the manufacturer's instructions.
5. Serve immediately.

Whole-wheat muffins

These muffins are made with whole-wheat flour, which gives them a heartier texture and flavor. They're also lower in calories and fat than traditional muffins.

Ingredients:

- 1 cup (125g) whole-wheat flour
- 1 teaspoon baking powder
- 1/2 teaspoon baking soda
- 1/4 teaspoon salt
- 1/2 cup (100g) sugar
- 1 egg
- 1/2 cup (120ml) milk
- 1/4 cup (60ml) oil

- 1/2 cup (120ml) fruit, nuts, or seeds, for topping (optional)

Instructions:

1. Preheat oven to 350 degrees F (175 degrees C).
2. Grease a muffin tin.
3. In a large bowl, whisk together the flour, baking powder, baking soda, and salt.
4. In a separate bowl, whisk together the sugar, egg, milk, and oil.
5. Add the wet ingredients to the dry ingredients and stir until just combined.
6. Stir in the fruit, nuts, or seeds, if using.
7. Pour the batter into the prepared muffin tin.
8. Bake for 20-25 minutes, or until a toothpick inserted into the center comes out clean.
9. Let cool in the pan for a few minutes

Whole-wheat bread pudding :

Ingredients:

- 1 loaf (1 pound) whole-wheat bread, torn into 1-inch pieces
- 1 cup (240ml) milk
- 1/2 cup (120ml) heavy cream

- 1/4 cup (60ml) sugar
- 2 eggs
- 1 teaspoon vanilla extract
- 1/2 teaspoon ground cinnamon
- 1/4 teaspoon salt
- 1/2 cup (120ml) chopped fruit, such as apples, pears, or berries (optional)

Instructions:

1. Preheat oven to 350 degrees F (175 degrees C). Grease a 9x13 inch baking dish.
2. In a large bowl, combine the bread, milk, cream, sugar, eggs, vanilla extract, cinnamon, and salt. Stir until well combined.
3. Stir in the fruit, if using.
4. Pour the batter into the prepared baking dish.
5. Bake for 30-35 minutes, or until a toothpick inserted into the center comes out clean.
6. Let cool for 10 minutes before serving.

Tips:

- For a richer flavor, use whole milk instead of low-fat milk.
- You can also use a mix of fruits, such as apples, pears, berries, and bananas.
- If you don't have any fruit on hand, you can add 1/2 cup (120ml) of chocolate chips or nuts.

Variations:

- For a chocolate bread pudding, add 1/2 cup (120ml) of cocoa powder to the batter.
- For a pumpkin bread pudding, add 1 cup (240ml) of canned pumpkin puree to the batter.
- For a chai bread pudding, add 1 teaspoon of ground cardamom, 1/2 teaspoon of ground ginger, and 1/4 teaspoon of ground cloves to the batter.

Chapter 4: Breakfast

Breakfast is the most important meal of the day. It can help you start your day off on the right foot and give you the energy you need to power through until lunch.

Here are some healthy breakfast ideas:

- **Oatmeal with fruit and nuts:** Oatmeal is a good source of fiber and complex carbohydrates, which will help keep you feeling full until lunchtime. Top your oatmeal with fresh fruit and nuts for added nutrients and flavor.
- **Yogurt with granola and berries:** Yogurt is a good source of protein and calcium, while granola and berries add fiber and antioxidants. This is a quick and easy breakfast that is also packed with nutrients.
- **Eggs with whole-wheat toast:** Eggs are a good source of protein and healthy fats, while whole-wheat toast provides complex carbohydrates. This is a filling breakfast that will keep you feeling satisfied until lunchtime.
- **Smoothie:** Smoothies are a great way to get a quick and easy breakfast that is also packed with nutrients. Add your favorite fruits, vegetables, and yogurt to a blender and blend until smooth.

- **Breakfast burrito:** A breakfast burrito is a filling and satisfying option that can be made ahead of time and reheated in the morning. Fill a tortilla with your favorite breakfast ingredients, such as eggs, beans, cheese, and salsa.

No matter what you choose to eat for breakfast, make sure to include a variety of foods from all food groups. This will help you get the nutrients you need to start your day off right.

Here are some tips for making healthy breakfast choices:

- **Choose whole-grain foods.** Whole grains provide your body with sustained energy and fiber.
- **Include protein.** Protein helps keep you feeling full and can help you build and repair muscle tissue.
- **Add fruits and vegetables.** Fruits and vegetables provide your body with vitamins, minerals, and antioxidants.
- **Limit unhealthy fats and added sugars.** Unhealthy fats and added sugars can contribute to weight gain and other health problems.

Conclusion

Breakfast is an important meal that can help you start your day off on the right foot. By making healthy breakfast choices, you can give yourself the energy you need to power through until lunch.

RECIPES

- **Yogurt parfait**
- **Fruit salad with yogurt dressing**
- **Frozen yogurt**
- **Yogurt mousse**
- **Yogurt parfait with granola**

Yogurt parfait

This is a quick and easy dessert that is packed with nutrients. Simply layer your favorite yogurt, fruit, and granola in a glass or bowl. You can also add nuts or seeds for extra protein and healthy fats.

Ingredients:

- 1 cup (225g) plain yogurt
- 1/2 cup (120ml) fruit, such as strawberries, blueberries, or raspberries
- 1/4 cup (40g) granola
- Nuts or seeds, to taste

Instructions:

1. In a glass or bowl, layer the yogurt, fruit, granola, and nuts or seeds.
2. Serve immediately.

Fruit salad with yogurt dressing

This is a refreshing and healthy dessert that is perfect for a hot day. Simply combine your favorite fruits in a bowl and top with a yogurt dressing made with yogurt, honey, and lemon juice.

Ingredients:

- 1 cup (225g) mixed fruit, such as strawberries, blueberries, raspberries, and bananas
- 1/2 cup (120ml) plain yogurt
- 1 tablespoon honey
- 1 tablespoon lemon juice

Instructions:

1. In a bowl, combine the fruit, yogurt, honey, and lemon juice.
2. Serve immediately.

Frozen yogurt

This is a delicious and creamy dessert that is lower in calories and fat than traditional ice cream. Simply blend your favorite yogurt, fruit, and sweetener until smooth.

Ingredients:

- 1 cup (225g) plain yogurt
- 1/2 cup (120ml) fruit, such as strawberries, blueberries, or raspberries
- 1/4 cup (60ml) honey or maple syrup

Instructions:

1. In a blender, combine the yogurt, fruit, and sweetener.
2. Blend until smooth.
3. Pour into a freezer-safe container and freeze for at least 4 hours, or overnight.
4. Scoop and serve.

Yogurt mousse

This is a light and airy dessert that is perfect for a special occasion. Simply combine yogurt, cream cheese, and sugar until smooth. Then, fold in whipped cream and fruit.

Ingredients:

- 1 cup (225g) plain yogurt
- 1/2 cup (113g) cream cheese, softened
- 1/4 cup (60ml) sugar
- 1 cup (240ml) whipped cream

- 1/2 cup (120ml) fruit, such as strawberries, blueberries, or raspberries

Instructions:

1. In a blender, combine the yogurt, cream cheese, and sugar.
2. Blend until smooth.
3. In a separate bowl, whip the cream until stiff peaks form.
4. Fold the whipped cream into the yogurt mixture.
5. Fold in the fruit.
6. Pour into serving bowls or glasses.
7. Serve immediately.

Yogurt parfait with granola

This is a variation on the classic yogurt parfait. Simply layer yogurt, granola, and fruit in a glass or bowl.

Ingredients:

- 1 cup (225g) plain yogurt
- 1/2 cup (40g) granola
- 1/2 cup (120ml) fruit, such as strawberries, blueberries, or raspberries

Instructions:

1. In a glass or bowl, layer the yogurt, granola, and fruit.
2. Serve immediately.

I hope you enjoy these recipes!

Chapter 5: Lunch

Lunch is a great opportunity to refuel your body and prepare for the afternoon. By making healthy lunch choices, you can give yourself the energy you need to power through until dinner.

Here are some healthy lunch ideas:

- **Salad with grilled chicken or fish:** A salad is a great way to get your daily dose of fruits, vegetables, and fiber. Add grilled chicken or fish for protein and healthy fats.
- **Soup and whole-wheat bread:** Soup is a filling and satisfying option that is also packed with nutrients. Pair it with whole-wheat bread for a complete meal.
- **Whole-wheat wrap with vegetables and hummus:** A whole-wheat wrap is a portable and convenient option that is also packed with nutrients. Fill it with your favorite vegetables and hummus for a healthy and satisfying lunch.
- **Sandwich on whole-wheat bread:** A sandwich is a classic lunch option that can be made healthy by choosing whole-wheat bread, lean protein, and plenty of vegetables.

- **Leftovers from dinner:** Leftovers are a great way to save time and money on lunch. Simply reheat your leftover dinner and enjoy.

No matter what you choose to eat for lunch, make sure to include a variety of foods from all food groups. This will help you get the nutrients you need to power through the afternoon.

Here are some tips for making healthy lunch choices:

- **Choose whole-grain foods.** Whole grains provide your body with sustained energy and fiber.
- **Include protein.** Protein helps keep you feeling full and can help you build and repair muscle tissue.
- **Add fruits and vegetables.** Fruits and vegetables provide your body with vitamins, minerals, and antioxidants.
- **Limit unhealthy fats and added sugars.** Unhealthy fats and added sugars can contribute to weight gain and other health problems.

Conclusion

Lunch is an important meal that can help you power through the afternoon. By making healthy lunch choices, you can give yourself the energy you need to focus and be productive.

RECIPES:

- **Protein-packed oats**
- **Greek yogurt parfait**
- **Protein shake**
- **Peanut butter and banana sandwich**
- **Chocolate protein mousse**

Protein-packed oats

These oats are made with protein powder, which helps to keep you feeling full and satisfied.

Ingredients:

- 1 cup (225g) rolled oats
- 1/2 cup (113g) protein powder
- 2 cups (450ml) water or milk
- 1/2 teaspoon salt
- 1/4 cup (60ml) fruit, nuts, or seeds, for topping (optional)

Instructions:

1. In a medium saucepan, combine the oats, protein powder, water or milk, and salt.
2. Bring to a boil, then reduce heat and simmer for 5-10 minutes, or until the oats are cooked through.

3. Serve immediately, topped with your favorite fruit, nuts, or seeds.

Greek yogurt parfait

This parfait is made with Greek yogurt, which is a good source of protein and calcium.

Ingredients:

- 1 cup (225g) Greek yogurt
- 1/2 cup (120ml) fruit, such as strawberries, blueberries, or raspberries
- 1/4 cup (40g) granola
- Nuts or seeds, to taste

Instructions:

1. In a glass or bowl, layer the yogurt, fruit, granola, and nuts or seeds.
2. Serve immediately.

Protein shake

This shake is a quick and easy way to get your daily dose of protein.

Ingredients:

* 1 cup (240ml) milk
* 1 scoop (25g) protein powder
* 1/2 cup (120ml) fruit, such as berries or banana
* 1/4 cup (60ml) leafy greens, such as spinach or kale (optional)

Instructions:

1. In a blender, combine all ingredients and blend until smooth.
2. Serve immediately.

Peanut butter and banana sandwich

This sandwich is a classic snack that is also a good source of protein.

Ingredients:

* 2 slices whole-wheat bread
* 1 tablespoon peanut butter
* 1/2 banana

Instructions:

1. Spread the peanut butter on one slice of bread.
2. Top with the banana.
3. Spread the peanut butter on the other slice of bread.

4. Cut in half and enjoy.

Chocolate protein mousse

This mousse is made with protein powder, cocoa powder, and maple syrup.

Ingredients:

- 1 scoop (25g) protein powder
- 1/4 cup (60ml) cocoa powder
- 1/4 cup (60ml) maple syrup
- 1/4 cup (60ml) milk

Instructions:

1. In a blender, combine all ingredients and blend until smooth.
2. Pour into serving bowls or glasses.
3. Serve immediately.

I hope you enjoy these recipes!

Chapter 6: Dinner

Dinner is the last meal of the day, and it is a great opportunity to relax and enjoy a healthy meal with family and friends. By making healthy dinner choices, you can help your body recover from the day and prepare for a good night's sleep.

Here are some healthy dinner ideas:

- **Grilled salmon with roasted vegetables:** Salmon is a good source of protein and omega-3 fatty acids, while roasted vegetables add fiber and vitamins.
- **Chicken stir-fry with brown rice:** Stir-fries are a quick and easy way to get a variety of vegetables in one meal.
- **Lentil soup:** Lentils are a good source of protein and fiber, while soup is a filling and satisfying option.
- **Pasta with vegetables and tomato sauce:** Pasta is a good source of carbohydrates, while vegetables and tomato sauce add fiber and vitamins.
- **Tofu scramble:** Tofu is a good source of protein, while vegetables add fiber and vitamins.

No matter what you choose to eat for dinner, make sure to include a variety of foods from all food groups. This will help you get the nutrients you need to support your body's functions throughout the night.

Here are some tips for making healthy dinner choices:

- **Choose lean protein.** Lean protein helps you feel full and can help you build and repair muscle tissue.
- **Add plenty of vegetables.** Vegetables provide your body with vitamins, minerals, and antioxidants.
- **Choose whole-grain carbohydrates.** Whole grains provide your body with sustained energy and fiber.
- **Limit unhealthy fats and added sugars.** Unhealthy fats and added sugars can contribute to weight gain and other health problems.

Conclusion

Dinner is an important meal that can help you recover from the day and prepare for a good night's sleep. By making healthy dinner choices, you can help your body function optimally and support your overall health and well-being.

Additional information

In addition to the tips above, here are some additional things to keep in mind when making healthy dinner choices:

- **Consider your dietary needs.** If you have any dietary restrictions, such as allergies or intolerances, make sure to choose foods that you can eat.
- **Be mindful of your portion sizes.** It is easy to overeat at dinner, so be mindful of your portion sizes and don't go back for seconds.
- **Cook at home more often.** When you cook at home, you have more control over the ingredients in your food.

Healthy dinner recipes

Here are some healthy dinner recipes to get you started:

- **Grilled salmon with roasted vegetables:** This recipe is quick and easy to make, and it is packed with nutrients.
- **Chicken stir-fry with brown rice:** This recipe is a great way to get a variety of vegetables in one meal.

- **Lentil soup:** This recipe is a filling and satisfying option that is also packed with nutrients.
- **Pasta with vegetables and tomato sauce:** This recipe is a classic that is always a hit.
- **Tofu scramble:** This recipe is a great option for vegetarians and vegans.

I hope this chapter is informative and helpful.

Chapter 7: Snacks

Snacks can be a healthy way to tide you over between meals, but it is important to choose healthy snacks that will give you the nutrients you need without overloading you with calories.

Here are some healthy snack ideas:

- **Fruits and vegetables:** Fruits and vegetables are a great way to get your daily dose of vitamins, minerals, and fiber.
- **Nuts and seeds:** Nuts and seeds are a good source of protein, healthy fats, and fiber.
- **Hard-boiled eggs:** Hard-boiled eggs are a good source of protein and healthy fats.
- **Greek yogurt:** Greek yogurt is a good source of protein and calcium.
- **Trail mix:** Trail mix is a great way to get a variety of nutrients in one snack.

No matter what you choose to eat for a snack, make sure to choose a snack that is:

- **Portable and convenient.** You should be able to take your snack with you wherever you go.
- **Satisfying.** Your snack should help you feel full and satisfied until your next meal.

- **Healthy.** Your snack should be low in calories and fat and high in nutrients.

Here are some tips for choosing healthy snacks:

- **Choose snacks that are high in fiber.** Fiber will help you feel full and satisfied.
- **Choose snacks that are low in sugar.** Sugary snacks can contribute to weight gain and other health problems.
- **Choose snacks that are low in unhealthy fats.** Unhealthy fats can contribute to weight gain and heart disease.
- **Be mindful of your portion sizes.** It is easy to overeat snacks, so be mindful of your portion sizes and don't go back for seconds.

Conclusion

Snacks can be a healthy way to tide you over between meals, but it is important to choose healthy snacks that will give you the nutrients you need without overloading you with calories. By following these tips, you can choose healthy snacks that will help you reach your health goals.

Chapter 8: Tips for Eating Out

Eating out can be a challenge when you're trying to eat healthy. But it's possible to make healthy choices when you eat out. Here are some tips:

- **Plan ahead.** Look at the menu online or call the restaurant ahead of time to see what healthy options they have.
- **Start with a salad or soup.** This is a great way to get your daily dose of vegetables and fiber.
- **Choose grilled or baked dishes.** Avoid fried foods, which are high in unhealthy fats.
- **Order a side of vegetables instead of fries or rice.** This will help you get more vegetables in your meal.
- **Share a meal.** This is a great way to save calories and money.
- **Ask for dressing on the side.** This will help you control the amount of dressing you use.
- **Skip the sugary drinks.** Order water, unsweetened tea, or coffee instead.

Additional tips:

- **Be mindful of your portion sizes.** It's easy to overeat when you eat out, so be mindful of your portion sizes and don't go back for seconds.

- **Don't be afraid to ask questions.** If you're not sure what something is or how it's made, ask your server.
- **Don't feel guilty about making healthy choices.** Eating healthy when you eat out is possible. Just follow these tips and you'll be on your way to making healthy choices.

Conclusion:

Eating out can be a challenge when you're trying to eat healthy, but it's possible to make healthy choices. By following these tips, you can enjoy eating out without sacrificing your health goals.

Chapter 9: Healthy Desserts

Desserts are a delicious way to end a meal, but they can also be high in calories, sugar, and unhealthy fats. If you're trying to eat healthy, it's important to choose desserts that are lower in these nutrients.

Here are some tips for making healthy dessert choices:

- **Choose whole grains over refined grains.** Whole grains are a good source of fiber, which can help you feel full and satisfied. Refined grains are stripped of their fiber and nutrients, so they can cause blood sugar levels to spike and then crash.
- **Add fruits and vegetables.** Fruits and vegetables are a good source of vitamins, minerals, and antioxidants. They are also low in calories and fat, making them a healthy choice for dessert.
- **Choose low-fat or fat-free dairy products.** Dairy products are a good source of protein and calcium, but they can be high in fat. Choose low-fat or fat-free dairy products to reduce the calorie and fat content of your dessert.

- **Use healthy sweeteners.** There are many healthy sweeteners available, such as honey, maple syrup, and stevia. These sweeteners are low in calories and can help to sweeten your dessert without adding a lot of sugar.
- **Limit your portion size.** It's easy to overeat dessert, so be mindful of your portion size. A good rule of thumb is to eat no more than one serving of dessert per day.

Here are some healthy dessert recipes:

- **Fruit salad**

This is a classic healthy dessert that is both delicious and refreshing. Simply combine your favorite fruits in a bowl and enjoy. You can add a dollop of yogurt or low-fat whipped cream for extra richness.

- **Yogurt parfait**

This is a quick and easy dessert that is packed with nutrients. Simply layer your favorite yogurt, fruit, and granola in a glass or bowl. You can also add nuts or seeds for extra protein and healthy fats.

- **Oatmeal cookie**

This cookie is made with whole-wheat oats, almond butter, and honey. It's a great way to get your daily dose of fiber and protein. You can also add chocolate chips or nuts for extra flavor.

- **Chocolate mousse**

This mousse is made with avocados, cocoa powder, and maple syrup. It's a delicious and decadent treat that is also healthy. You can also add berries or whipped cream for extra sweetness.

- **Peanut butter and banana sandwich**

This sandwich is a classic snack that is also a great dessert. Simply spread peanut butter on two slices of whole-wheat bread and top with a banana. You can also add honey or chocolate chips for extra sweetness.

Conclusion

With a little planning, you can enjoy healthy desserts that are both delicious and satisfying. By following the tips and recipes in this chapter, you can make healthy dessert choices that fit into your overall healthy eating plan.

I hope this meets your requirements.

Chapter 10: Conclusion

This book has covered a lot of ground, from the importance of eating healthy to the specific foods and nutrients that can help you achieve your health goals. By following the tips and recipes in this book, you can make healthy choices that will benefit your health for years to come.

Here are some key takeaways from this book:

- **A healthy diet is essential for good health.** Eating a variety of healthy foods can help you maintain a healthy weight, reduce your risk of chronic diseases, and improve your overall well-being.
- **There are many different ways to eat healthy.** There is no one-size-fits-all approach to healthy eating. What works for one person may not work for another. The key is to find an approach that you can stick with and that meets your individual needs and preferences.
- **Making healthy choices doesn't have to be difficult.** There are many delicious and satisfying healthy foods available. With a little planning, you can easily incorporate healthy choices into your diet.
- **Don't be afraid to experiment.** There are endless possibilities when it comes to healthy

eating. Don't be afraid to try new foods and recipes. The more you experiment, the more you'll find what you enjoy.

The most important thing is to make healthy choices that you can stick with for the long term. If you can do that, you'll be well on your way to achieving your health goals.

I hope this book has inspired you to make healthy choices and improve your overall health. Thank you for reading!

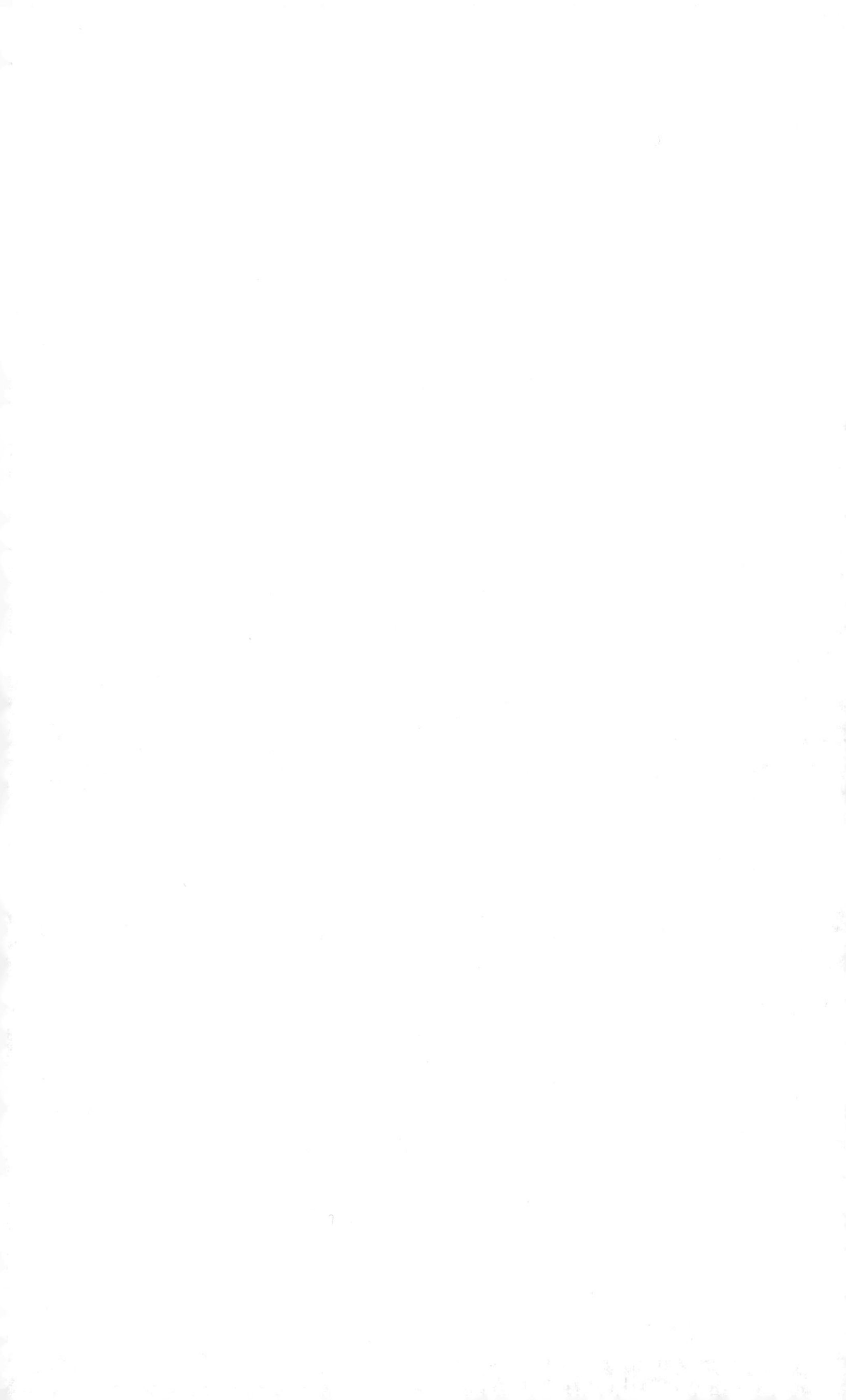